GINKGO BILOBA

MARIAN KIM

CONTENTS

MARIAN KIM

1

PROPERTIES

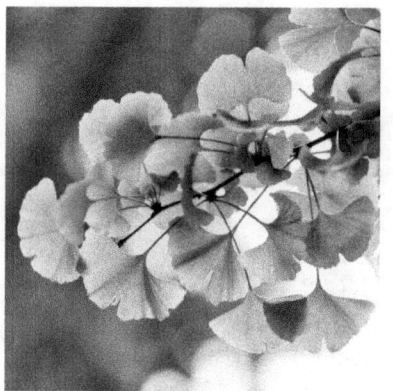

Scientific name: Ginkgo biloba

Other names: Maidenhair tree, fossil tree, kew tree, bai guo

Properties

Antioxidant properties which protect the cells from the free radical damage that causes premature aging and degenerative diseases.

Antiaging properties

Anti-inflammatory properties

Anticancer properties

Antidepressant properties

Antihistamine properties

Antitussive (reduces coughing) properties

Astringent properties

* * * * *

2

USES

Depression treatment

Ginkgo biloba has a mild stimulatory effect on the brain and it increases blood flow to the brain. It has therefore been used to manage winder depression in persons with seasonal affective disorder (SAD). Doses for depression are around 80 mg three times a day.

Alzheimer's disease

Ginkgo biloba is used for Alzheimer's disease. Some studies suggest that taking ginkgo leaf extract can improve the symptoms of Alzheimer's disease and other forms of dementia.

Age related brain disorders

Ginkgo biloba is used to improve thinking skills in persons with thinking problems caused by old age. It also acts as a memory booster and improves memory in age related memory loss.

Ginkgo is also used for brain health in elderly persons with conditions thought to be caused by reduced blood flow in the brain. These conditions include vertigo, tinnitus (ringing in the ears), headache, difficulty concentrating and mood disorders.

Improve thinking

Ginkgo biloba leaf extract is used to improve cognitive functions like thinking, the speed of mental processing and memory in healthy persons without memory loss.

Claudication treatment

Ginkgo biloba is used to treat claudication which is a condition that causes pain in the legs when walking due to poor blood flow.

Some studies show that taking gingko can increase the distance that persons with this condition can walk without experiencing pain.

Raynaud's syndrome treatment

Ginkgo biloba is used to treat Raynaud's phenomenon which is a condition associated with poor circulation in which the fingers and toes change color when it is cold and become painful.

Ginkgo leaf extract has been shown to reduce the number of painful attacks in persons with Raynaud's syndrome.

Vertigo and dizziness treatment

Ginkgo biloba leaf has been shown to improve dizziness and vertigo.

Glaucoma treatment

Ginkgo biloba is used to improve damage to the visual field in persons with normal tension (pressure) glaucoma.

Taking the leaf extract has also been shown to improve color vision in persons whose eyes have been damaged by diabetes.

Premenstrual syndrome (PMS) management

Ginkgo biloba is used for PMS. The leaf extract is taken orally to reduce PMS symptoms like breast pain when it is taken from day 16 of the cycle to day 5 of the next cycle.

Altitude sickness prevention

Ginkgo biloba is used to prevent mountain or altitude sickness in climbers.

Allergy treatment

Ginkgo biloba is used to relieve the congestion of allergies.

Aphrodisiac

Ginkgo biloba is used for sexual performance disorders since it increases blood flow in the genital area in both men and women. It is also used to treat those which develop as a result of taking antidepressants.

Bruises and burns treatment

Ginkgo biloba poultice is used to help mild bruises and burns heal.

Cellulite treatment

Ginkgo biloba is used to treat cellulite.

Detoxification

Ginkgo biloba is used for detoxification.

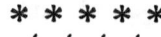

* * * * *

3

SAFETY PRECAUTIONS

1. Women who are pregnant should not use/avoid ginkgo biloba since it can cause premature (early) labor or excessive bleeding during delivery.

2. Persons with diabetes should not use/avoid ginkgo biloba since it can interfere with the control of blood sugar levels.

3. Persons with seizure disorders should not use/avoid ginkgo biloba since it can cause seizures (convulsions).

4. Persons with infertility should not use/avoid ginkgo biloba since it can interfere getting pregnant.

5. Persons with bleeding disorders should not use/avoid ginkgo biloba since it can worsen the disorder.

6. Persons scheduled to have surgery should not use for at least 2 weeks before the scheduled operation since it can cause bleeding during or after surgery.

GINKGO BILOBA

*, *, *, *

4

DRUG INTERACTIONS

1. Persons using blood thinners like coumadin (Warfarin), heparin, aspirin and other antiplatelet medications like clopidogrel (Plavix), dalteparin (Fragmin), enoxaparin (Lovenox) should avoid/not use gingko biloba since it can slow blood clotting and lead to bleeding. Other medications that can also slow blood clotting include diclofenac (Voltrare, Cataflam) and ibuprofen (Motrin, Advil).

2. Persons taking alprazolam (Xanax) should avoid using/not use gingko biloba since it can decrease the effects of alprazolam.

3. Persons taking efavirenz (Sustiva) which is used to treat HIV should avoid using/not use gingko biloba since it can decrease the effects of efavirenz.

4. Persons taking fluoxetine (Prozac) should avoid using/not use gingko biloba since it can cause hypomania and make them feel nervous.

5. Persons taking medications changed by the liver should avoid using/not use gingko biloba since it can decrease how quickly they are

broken down and increase their effects and side effects. Examples of these medications include haloperidol (Haldol), imipramine (Tofranil), propranolol (Inderal) and theophylline.

Gingko can also increase how quickly some medications are broken down and decrease their effects. Examples of these medications include amitriptyline (Elavil), citalopram (Celexa), diazepam (Valium), omeprazole (Prilosec), phenytoin (Dilantin) and warfarin (Coumadin).

6. Persons using diabetes medications should avoid using/not use gingko biloba since it can decrease or increase insulin levels and blood glucose levels in persons with type 2 diabetes.

7. Persons using anticonvulsants or medications to prevent seizures should avoid using/not use gingko biloba since it can decrease their effectiveness. Examples of these anticonvulsants include phenytoin (Dilantin), carbamazepine (Tegretol), valproic acid (Depakene), gabapentin (Neurontin) and phenobarbital.

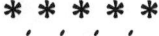

5

HERBAL RECIPES

Ginkgo Tea

Equipment
Tea pot or kettle

***

Ingredients
1 teaspoon of dried ginkgo leaves

1 cup of boiling water

Honey to taste (optional)

***

Instructions

1. Put the ginkgo in a tea pot or kettle, add the boiling water and let it steep while covered for 10 -15 minutes.

2. Add honey (if using) to suit your taste before drinking.

*****

Ginkgo Infusion

Equipment
Glass jar with tight fitting lid

***

Ingredients
1 teaspoon dried ginkgo

1 cup boiling water

***

Instructions
1. Place the ginkgo in the glass jar and add the boiling water.

2. Close the lid and let the mixture steep for 4 hours to 14 hours (overnight).

3. Strain the ginkgo and the infusion is ready for consumption as ginkgo tea.

4. Store the infusion in the refrigerator to lengthen its life.

*****

Ginkgo Syrup

Equipment

Saucepan

Jar with airtight lid

***

Ingredients

1 quart (1000 ml) filtered water

1 cup dried ginkgo leaves

1 cup honey

***

Instructions

1. Place the water and ginkgo in a saucepan and bring to a boil.

2. Reduce the heat and let it simmer while it is partially covered until the volume is reduced to half the original volume.

3. Strain the mixture through a sieve or cheesecloth to remove the ginkgo.

4. Measure 1 pint (500 ml) of the liquid and add the honey.

5. Cook for a few minutes as you stir it so that it thickens.

6. Store the syrup in an airtight container in the fridge for up to 2 months.

***

Tips

1. Make this syrup more potent for relieving coughs by adding herbs and spices like ginger and lemon balm.

*****

Ginkgo Tincture

Equipment

Glass jar with tight fitting lid

Dark tincture bottles

Cheesecloth

Labels

***

Ingredients

7 oz (200 gm) of dried ginkgo

30 oz (1 liter) of 80-100 proof vodka

***

Instructions

1. Fill 1/3 of the glass jar with the ginkgo.

2. Add the vodka to completely fill the jar to the top.

3. Seal the jar and label it with the date of preparation and name of botanical (ginkgo) used.

4. Store the glass jar in a dark place for 6 weeks ensuring that you shake them weekly.

5. After 6 weeks strain out the ginkgo with a cheesecloth and pour the tincture into dark tincture bottles.

6. Label the tincture bottles with the date and name of botanical (ginkgo) used.

7. Store your herbal tinctures away from light and heat.

*****

Ginkgo Poultice

Equipment
Cheesecloth or old cotton sheet strips

***

Ingredients
1 tablespoon crushed fresh ginkgo leaves

Boiling water

***

Instructions
1. Add enough boiling water to the ginkgo to wet it and make a thick paste.

2. Spoon the ginkgo paste onto the cheesecloth (or bed sheet strips) to make the poultice.

3. To use, apply the poultice to the affected area and cover with another piece of hot, wet cloth. Replace the hot, wet cloth when it cools with another hot one to keep the poultice hot.

###

ABOUT THE AUTHOR

Marian Kim is an experienced alternative medicine practitioner.

OTHER BOOKS BY THE AUTHOR

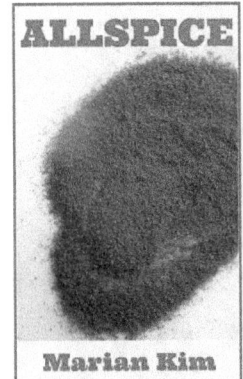
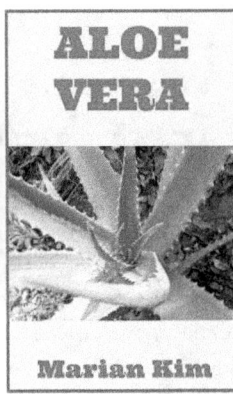
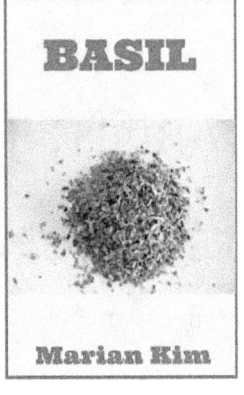
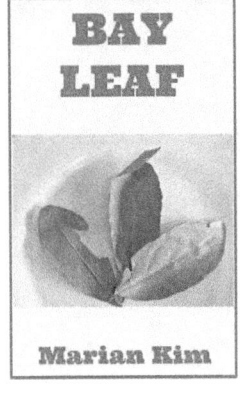
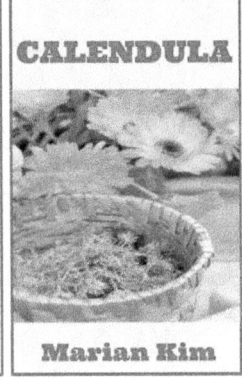
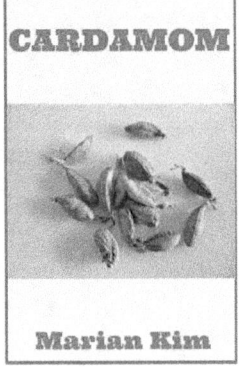

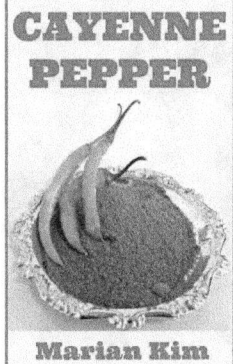

CAYENNE PEPPER

Marian Kim

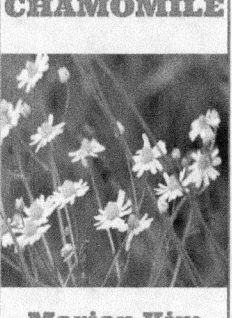

CHAMOMILE

Marian Kim

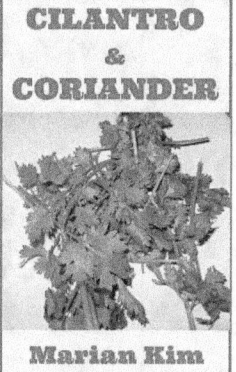

CILANTRO & CORIANDER

Marian Kim

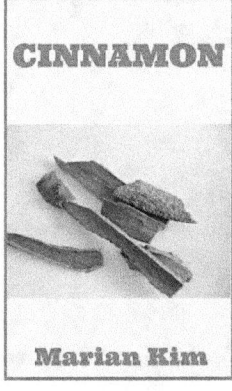

CINNAMON

Marian Kim

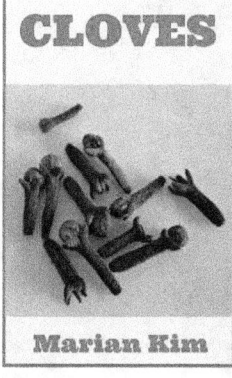

CLOVES

Marian Kim

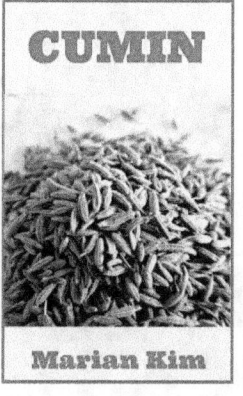

CUMIN

Marian Kim

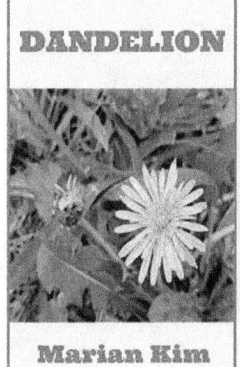

DANDELION

Marian Kim

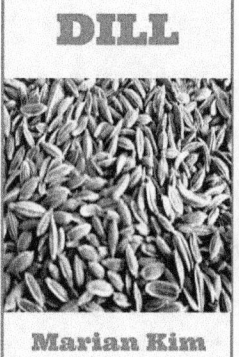

DILL

Marian Kim

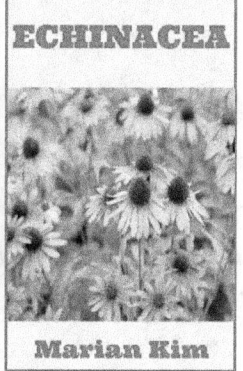

ECHINACEA

Marian Kim

FENNEL
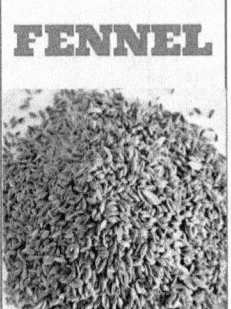
Marian Kim

FENUGREEK
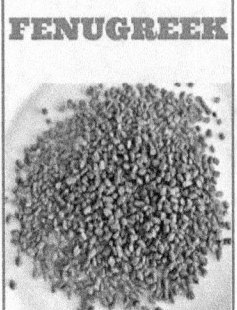
Marian Kim

GARLIC
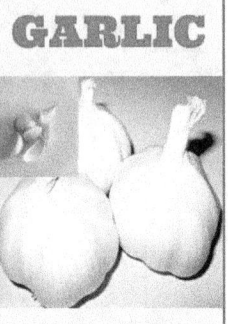
Marian Kim

GINGER
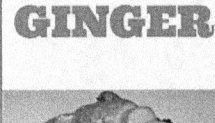
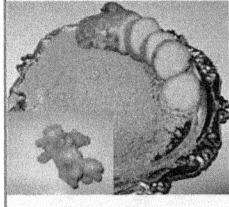
Marian Kim

GINKGO BILOBA
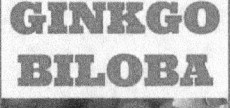
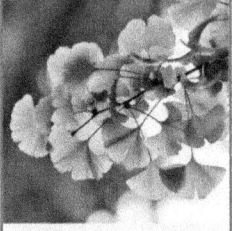
Marian Kim

GINSENG
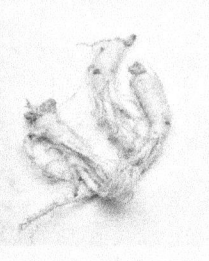
Marian Kim

LAVENDER
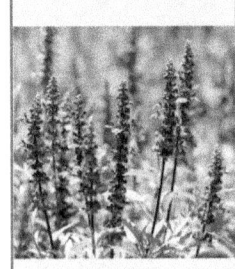
Marian Kim

MUSTARD
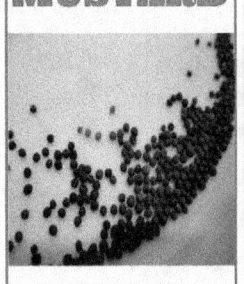
Marian Kim

NEEM
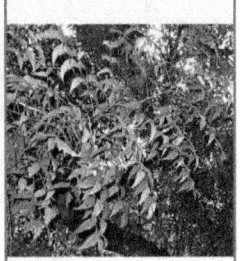
Marian Kim

NUTMEG & MACE
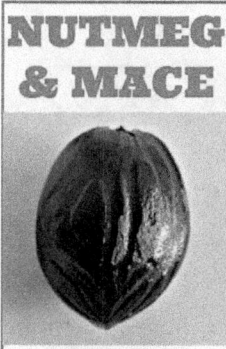
Marian Kim

OREGANO
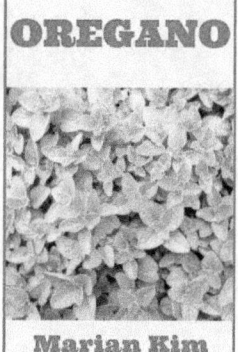
Marian Kim

PAPRIKA
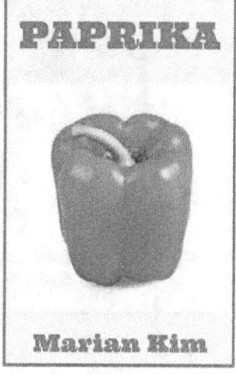
Marian Kim

PARSLEY
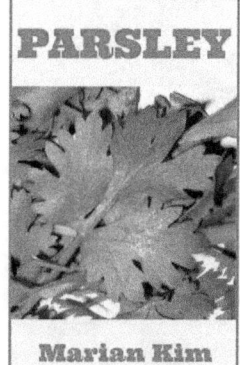
Marian Kim

BLACK & WHITE PEPPER
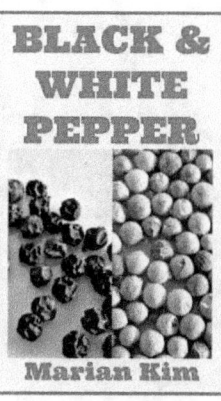
Marian Kim

PEPPERMINT
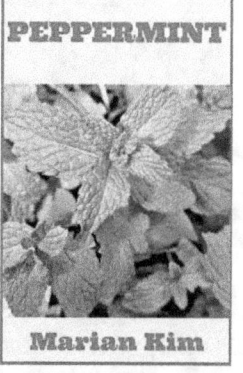
Marian Kim

ROSE HIPS
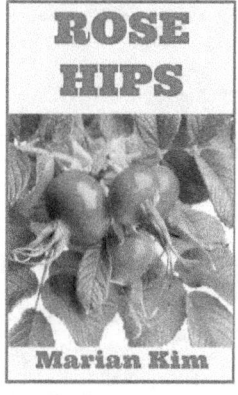
Marian Kim

ROSE PETALS
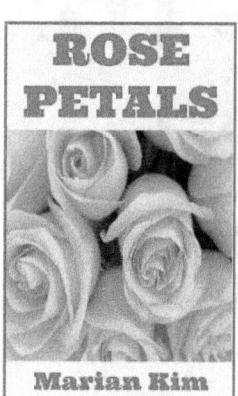
Marian Kim

ROSEMARY
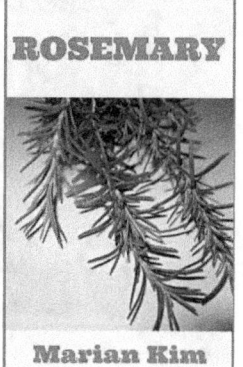
Marian Kim

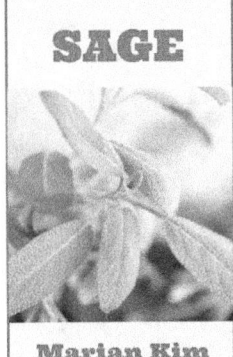

SAGE

Marian Kim

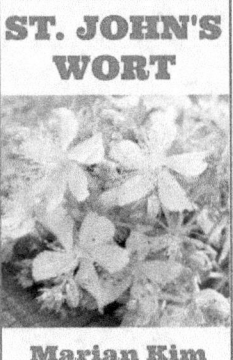

ST. JOHN'S WORT

Marian Kim

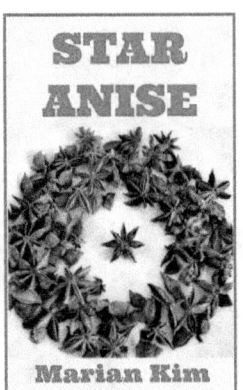

STAR ANISE

Marian Kim

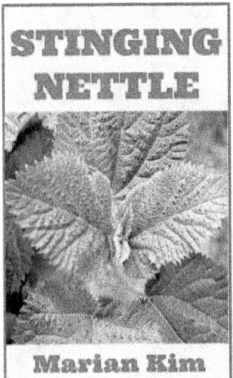

STINGING NETTLE

Marian Kim

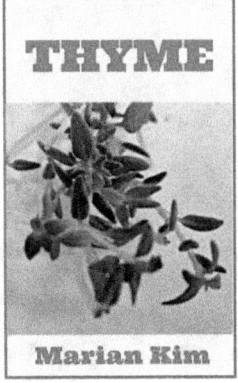

THYME

Marian Kim

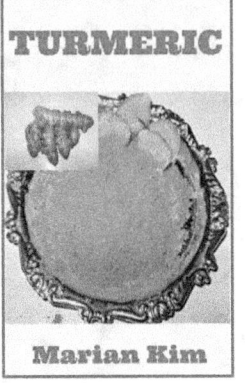

TURMERIC

Marian Kim

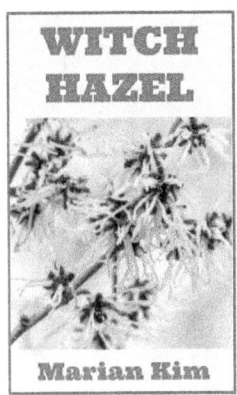

WITCH HAZEL

Marian Kim

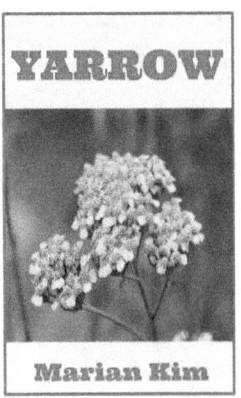

YARROW

Marian Kim

*****

www.ingramcontent.com/pod-product-compliance
Lightning Source LLC
Chambersburg PA
CBHW071348310526
45790CB00018B/1393